Dr. Mom

Ten Top Tips
for the Health *and* Safety
of Your Child

Dr. Mom: Ten Top Tips for the Health and Safety of Your Child covers the scope of need-to-know information with logical, sensible and easily accomplished advice presented by the father/daughter team of Catherine Dilts Carter, RN, CPNP and Preston V. Dilts, Jr., MD., based on their research with 14 prominent physicians. Read, learn and use the checklists to chart your progress.

Other Books from

Inside Advantage Publications

Sleep Disorders:
America's Hidden Nightmare

One Step Ahead:
The Unused Keys to Success

Bounce Back and Win:
What It Takes and How To Do It

Fast Track:
How To Gain and Keep Momentum

Magnet People:
Their Secrets and How to Learn from Them

Little Things, Big Results –
How Small Events Determine Our Fate

How to Recognize Substance Abuse:
At Work, at Home, in Athletics… Anywhere

To Order: phone (630) 420-7673; fax (630) 420-7835;
e-mail: RFritz3800@aol.com;
webpage: www.rogerfritz.com

Dr. Mom

Ten Top Tips
for the Health *and* Safety
of Your Child

by

Catherine Dilts Carter, RN, CPNP
and
Preston V. Dilts, Jr., MD

Inside Advantage Publications
Naperville, Illinois

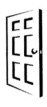

Published by:
Inside Advantage Publications
1240 Iroquois Drive, Suite 406
Naperville, IL 60563
Phone: 630.420.7673
Fax: 630.420.7835
rfritz3800@aol.com
http://www.rogerfritz.com

Cover and Book Design by Charles King

1-893987-07-8

http://www.rogerfritz.com

Inside Advantage Publications
Naperville, Illinois

Introduction

WHEN WE FIRST BEGAN to work on a 'Ten Top Tips' survey, we were inundated with ideas from our experts far beyond our imaginations. Tabulating them to arrive at a vote for the top ten proved impossible. So we have selected the ten top categories into which we have condensed the most frequent suggestions for health and safety. A chapter is devoted to each. As a summary for each chapter, we've provided a checklist of suggestions and a quick way to chart your progress. There is some repetition of topics we believe are especially significant.

Nothing is more important to a parent than the health and safety of their children. Children are precious gifts. Protecting and nurturing them is life's greatest challenge and satisfaction. With all the information available through the media (print, TV and radio) and the Internet, it's hard to choose the best resources — ones you can trust. We want 'Ten Top Tips' to be high on that list.

No book or list of tips can possibly replace the advice and expertise of your health care practitioner who has direct contact with you and your child. *Dr. Mom: Ten Top Tips for Health and Safety of your Child* is not intended to do so. We hope our suggestions will lead you to consult your health care practitioner more effectively, which should lead to greater understanding of problems and how to avoid them. Suggestions are always welcome.

Notice to Readers

The authors, contributors, editor and publisher have gone to great effort to ensure that the recommendations made are accurate and in agreement with other authorities and national organizations. However, constant change and new information does and will occur. In addition, differences in opinion over common clinical situations do occasionally happen. We suggest you should always respect the suggestions of your health care provider if this should occur. Open discussion will lead to better understanding.

About the Authors

The authors bring the very unusual expertise of a father-daughter team with extensive and direct experience in childcare.

Catherine Dilts Carter is a Pediatric Nurse Practitioner, married, with a boy and a girl, ages 8 and 10. She graduated with a Bachelor of Science in Nursing from Vanderbilt University, Nashville, TN and a Master of Science from the University of Michigan, Ann Arbor, MI. She is certified by the National Board of Pediatric Nurse Practitioners and has practiced at Kid's Creek Children's Clinic in Traverse City, MI for fifteen years.

Her father, Preston V. Dilts, Jr., married, with three grown children and four grandchildren, graduated from Northwestern University Medical School, Chicago, IL and received a Master of Science in Gynecologic Pathology from Northwestern University, Evanston, IL. He is certified by the American Board of Obstetrics and Gynecology and sub-specialty certified in Maternal-Fetal Medicine. He was chairman of the Departments of Obstetrics and Gynecology at the University of North Dakota Medical School, Grand Forks, ND, the University of Tennessee College of Medicine, Memphis, TN, and the University of Michigan Medical School, Ann Arbor, MI. He is Emeritus Professor of Obstetrics and Gynecology at the University of Missouri School of Medicine, Kansas City, MO. In addition, Dr. Dilts was a member of the Editorial Board and a contributor to *The Merck Manual* and the *Merck Manual of Medical Information*, Home Edition.

Acknowledgements

We decided to ask medical doctors from a variety of specialties in order to be sure we covered the whole scope of health and safety tips needed to protect your children. We have included a trauma surgeon, several pediatricians, several family practitioners, an obstetrician and a psychiatrist. They are:

Paul Antal, MD
    MD — Jefferson Medical College, Philadelphia, PA
    Certified American Board of Family Medicine
    Lake Shore Family Care, Manistee, MI

Matthew Boulis, MD
    MD — Jefferson Medical College, Philadelphia, PA
    Certified American Board Pediatrics
    Kids First/Cinnaminson Pediatrics, Cinnaminson, NJ

Pamela Bradt, MD, MPH
    MD — University of Kansas School of Medicine, Kansas City, KS
    MPH — University of Texas School of Public Health, Houston, TX
    Certified American Board of Pediatrics
    Assistant Professor University of Missouri School of Medicine, Kansas City
    General Pediatrician, Children's Mercy Hospital, Kansas City, MO

Stephen L. Dilts, MD, PhD.
MD — Northwestern University Medical School,
Chicago, IL
PhD — Northwestern University, Evanston, IL
Certified American Board of Psychiatry, General
Psychiatry and Addiction Psychiatry
Past President American Academy of Addiction
Psychiatry
Clinical Professor Psychiatry, University of
Colorado, Denver, CO

Michael J. Eldredge, MD, MS
MD — Wayne State University School of Medicine,
Detroit, MI
MS — University of Wisconsin, Madison, WI
Certified American Board of Pediatrics
Kids Creek Children's Clinic, Traverse City, MI

Karen A. Funk, MD
MD — University of Illinois College of Medicine,
Chicago, IL
Resident in Family Medicine, Rose Medical Center,
Denver, CO

Margaret M. Griffen, MD
MD — University of Kentucky College of Medicine,
Lexington, KY
Certified American Board of Surgery and Surgical
Critical Care
Assistant Professor of Surgery, University of Florida
College of Medicine at Jacksonville
Trauma Surgeon

Ward O. Griffen, Jr., MD, PhD
   MD — Cornell University Medical College, New
      York, NY
   PhD — University of Minnesota, Minneapolis, MN
   Certified American Board of Surgery and
      Thoracic Surgery
   Past Executive Director American Board of
      Surgery
   Professor of Surgery, University of Kentucky
      College of Medicine, Retired

Sheldon B. Korones, MD
   MD — University of Tennessee School of
      Medicine, Memphis, TN
   Certified American Board of Pediatrics
   Alumni Distinguished Service Professor of
      Pediatrics and Obstetrics and Gynecology,
      University of Tennessee College of Medicine,
      Memphis, TN
   Director Newborn Intensive Care Center,
      Regional Medical Center, Memphis, TN

David F. McNeeley, MD, MPHTM
   MD — Tulane University School of Medicine,
      New Orleans, LA
   MPHTM — Tulane University School of Public
      Health and Tropical Medicine, New Orleans, LA
   Certified American Board of Pediatrics and
      American Society of Tropical Medicine and
      Hygiene
   Assistant Professor of Pediatrics, Weill Medical
      College of Cornell University, New York, NY

Trent McNeeley, MD
    MD — University of Tennessee College of
        Medicine, Memphis, TN
    Certified American Board of Family Medicine
    McNeeley Family Physicians, Norris, TN

Karla M. Smith, MD
    MD — Indiana University School of Medicine,
        Indianapolis, IN
    Certified American Board of Pediatrics and
        Pediatric Pulmonology
    Kids Creek Children's Clinic, Traverse City, MI

Allan B. Weingold, MD
    MD — New York Medical College, New York,
        NY
    Certified American Board of Obstetrics and
        Gynecology and Maternal-Fetal Medicine
    Past Vice President for Medical Affairs and
        Executive Dean, The George Washington
        University, Washington, DC
    Oscar I. Dodek Professor of Obstetrics
        and Gynecology, Emeritus, The George
        Washington University, Washington, DC

Contents

Chapter 1
Mother Nature
Designed It Best

THE HUMAN BODY IS TRULY MARVELOUS. Women's bodies are designed perfectly for the growth, nurturing and nourishment of babies — both inside *and* outside the womb.

PRENATAL CARE

> *Prenatal care is one of the highest*
> *priorities for the health*
> *and safety of your child.*

Ideally you can anticipate, and make some healthful changes, before your pregnancy begins. For example, stop smoking. Stop use of alcohol. Stop any recreational drugs, *permanently*. Don't take any medicines unless they are prescribed by your doctor. Try to get your weight in order. Eat a well-balanced, nutritious diet. If you are diabetic, get your blood sugars under tight control and keep them that way. Begin prenatal vitamins which include iron and folic acid. See your obstetrician, family practitioner or nurse midwife for other helpful tips.

As soon as you have missed a period, see your health care provider to establish your due date and begin the process of preventive care. Be sure to attend prenatal and birthing classes, which will include breastfeeding. You should gain 30 to 35 lbs during your pregnancy unless advised otherwise. This will provide nourishment enough to allow proper growth of your baby and provide enough fat to support milk production. Exercise moderately throughout your pregnancy. Obviously, through all this, involve your mate as much as possible, especially in the prenatal classes. If they are offered, both of you should attend child rearing classes.

Dr. Allan Weingold urges that you discuss with and follow the suggestions of your health care provider for immunizations, Rh incompatibility screening, ultrasound exams, genetic testing, and blood pressure checks.

All help insure a healthy pregnancy, delivery and successful breastfeeding.

BREASTFEEDING

Dr. Karen Funk strongly believes that breastfeeding your baby certainly is the best way to go.

You should begin in the hospital immediately after delivery. Your milk will come in after three or four days and your baby will get plenty of nourishment until then from colostrum secreted by your breasts.

The American Academy of Pediatrics recommends breast milk for the entire first year of your baby's life.

We recommend breastfeeding for several reasons. First of all, mother nature really did design women's bodies to feed their babies. The closeness and warmth cannot be achieved in any other way. The only part missing is a way for dad to participate. Pumping your breasts to allow him to bottle feed your baby with breast milk will keep him involved. And, he can participate in all the other aspects of care. Second, it's becoming more and more apparent that babies were designed for breast milk only, as is evident especially as they grow older. The number of people with lactose intolerance from cow's milk is astonishing, and may be linked to its early introduction. Third, some limited immunity is passed from mother to baby through breast milk which helps prevent infections in the newborn period.

- Breastfeeding helps a new mother recover from childbirth, as hormones secreted during nursing help control bleeding from the uterus.
- Breastfeeding has been identified as having a mood elevating or antidepressant effect for post partum women.
- Breastfeeding has been linked with a lower incidence of allergies, respiratory infections, and ear infections in children.

- Some studies have suggested that breastfeeding is linked with higher IQ scores in children.
- It has been well documented that iron is more readily absorbed from breast milk than from prepared infant formulas, which reduces the risk of iron deficiency anemia in your infant.
- Once established, breastfeeding requires no preparation, no shopping, mixing, dish washing, or heating. A mother needs only herself and her baby.
- Breastfeeding is *free* — what a bargain!

Breastfeeding is one of mother nature's greatest gifts with so many benefits. Breastfeeding your baby may be one of the most natural and instinctive activities a new mother can do with and for her baby. Don't miss the opportunity!

CHECKLIST

Use this Checklist to track your progress in meeting the recommendations in this chapter.

Goal	Accomplished		Will do		By When
	Yes	No	Yes	No	Date
Stop smoking					
Stop alcohol while pregnant or nursing, and then only in moderation					
Stop drugs					
Take only prescribed medicines while pregnant or nursing					
Take prenatal vitamins with iron and folic acid					
See your health care provider early to establish your due date					
Attend prenatal classes, both Mom and Dad					
Attend birthing classes, both Mom and Dad					
Attend child rearing classes, both Mom and Dad					
Gain 30 to 35 lbs during pregnancy					
Exercise moderately during pregnancy					
Involve your mate in childbirth preparation					
Have appropriate screening and testing during pregnancy					
Breast feed your baby					
Pump so Dad may bottle feed					

Chapter 2
Prevention
Is the Best Medicine

THE FOCUS OF HEALTH CARE today is prevention of illness, early detection and intervention for problems. Here are several things parents can do to promote their child's health.

IMMUNIZATIONS

The childhood diseases we now vaccinate against used to be deadly, disabling and disfiguring. The key is *used to be*. We have the power to prevent these illnesses for our children through immunization.

Dr. Matthew Boulis, calls immunizations "truly one of the greatest accomplishments of science in the 19th and 20th centuries."

Dr. David McNeeley strongly urges all parents to: "Make sure your child receives all recommended immunizations."

In fact, **childhood immunizations were mentioned more frequently than any other tip from our panel of experts.**

There is a regular schedule of immunizations, beginning in the newborn period, recommended by the Centers for Disease Control and Prevention and the American Academy of Pediatrics. This schedule is constantly changing as research is done to increase effectiveness. Many diseases are prevented by childhood immunization, and others could be added in the near future.

Diphtheria is a bacterial infection spread from person to person by respiratory droplets causing a low grade fever and a severe throat infection which can lead to airway obstruction and death. This illness has virtually been wiped out by immunization. The initial series of vaccines is completed between the ages of 4 and 6 years, with booster doses given every ten years (in conjunction with Tetanus vaccine) throughout your life.

Tetanus is a bacterial infection which invades wounds and can lead to a life threatening neurologic condition commonly referred to as 'lockjaw.' Tetanus is found in soil and in animal and human fecal material. The initial series of vaccines is completed between the ages of 4 and 6 years, with booster doses given every ten years (with Diphtheria) throughout your life. Tetanus bacteria continue to exist in the environment, but immunization has greatly reduced the incidence of infection.

Pertussis (also known as **whooping cough**) is a bacterial infection spread from person to person by respiratory droplets. It causes apnea (cessation of breathing), spasmodic cough (or whoop), pneumonia, and, in its worst form, seizures, brain inflammation, and death. Pertussis infections have been significantly reduced by immunization. However, it still remains a threat to under or unimmunized children. Pertussis causes the equivalent of a severe cold in older adults whose immunity has waned since childhood. They can then pass it on to children who are not fully immunized. Several cases of pertussis in children occur each year in most communities and could be prevented by immunization. The series of vaccines for pertussis is completed between the ages of 4 and 6.

- **The DTaP vaccine immunizes against Diphtheria, Tetanus and Pertussis.**

<u>Polio</u> is a viral infection spread from person to person by oral contact or contact with fecal material or contaminated water. Polio can cause paralysis and residual nerve damage. Adults who had polio as children may suffer from post-polio syndrome, a progressive neurologic condition. Polio has been eradicated from North America and most of the world through almost universal immunization. The series of vaccines for polio is completed between the ages of 4 and 6.

<u>Hemophilus Influenza Type B (Hib)</u> causes a bacterial infection spread from person to person by respiratory droplets. It causes blood infection, meningitis and epiglottitis — each of which can be deadly in young children. Fifteen years ago, Hib disease caused the majority of hospitalizations in children. Hib also used to be the cause of the majority of ear infections. Today, the incidence of Hib disease is rare, due to the success of immunization. The series of vaccines for Hib is completed by 18 months.

- **The DTaP/Hib vaccine, given to toddlers as a booster, contains the Diphtheria, Tetanus, Pertussis and Hib vaccines.**

Hepatitis B (Hep B) is a viral infection which is spread from person to person through blood and body fluids, including saliva and sexual contact. It is becoming more prevalent and is more easily spread than the AIDS virus. Hep B causes inflammation of and possible destruction of the liver. It also causes an increased risk of liver cancer. **Hep B is thought to cause more deaths each year than AIDS.** Hep B is *not* under control and the hope is that immunization of today's children will lead to its control in the next generation. The series of vaccines against Hep B is completed by the age of 6 months.

- **The Hepatitis B vaccine may be given in a combined vaccine with Hib — (Hib/Hep).**

Pneumococcus causes a bacterial infection which is spread from person to person through respiratory droplets. It is currently the most common cause of meningitis and blood infections in infants. Pneumococcus also causes pneumonia and a majority of ear infections in children. Pneumococcal disease is a widespread risk and the vaccine was implemented for children only recently. Older adults and those with lung disease are also vulnerable to pneumococcal disease and an adult version of this vaccine is recommended for them. The series of vaccines against pneumococcus is completed by the age of 2.

Measles is a viral infection which is spread from person to person through respiratory droplets. It causes a high fever, a severe rash, and can be deadly if it progresses to encephalitis (brain inflammation). Measles has become very uncommon thanks to immunization. Rare outbreaks occur — usually in large cities or on college campuses where people from countries in which the disease is not controlled may be visiting. The series of vaccines against measles is completed between the ages of 4 and 6.

Mumps is a viral infection which is spread from person to person by respiratory droplets. It causes high fever and severe swelling of the salivary glands. Complications include deafness and sterility in males if the disease spreads. Mumps can also cause miscarriages in pregnant women. Mumps is rarely seen today thanks to the vaccine. The series of vaccines against mumps is completed between the ages of 4 and 6.

Rubella (German or 3 day measles) is a viral infection which is spread from person to person by respiratory droplets. It causes 3 days of rash in children. The largest risk from rubella is to the unborn child. When pregnant women contract rubella early in pregnancy it can cause birth defects including blindness in the newborn. Rubella is rare thanks to immunization and careful screening of immunity in women of childbearing age. The series of vaccines for rubella are completed between the ages of 4 and 6.

- **The MMR vaccine immunizes against Measles, Mumps and Rubella.**

Chicken pox (varicella zoster) is caused by a virus which is spread from person to person through respiratory droplets. It causes fever and an ulcer like rash which can leave scars. Complications include severe skin infection which can lead to disfiguring scarring, and meningitis and encephalitis which can be deadly. Adults who had chicken pox as a child can suffer from a reactivation of the virus (which continues to live in nerve roots) called 'shingles' or herpes zoster. The incidence of chicken pox has decreased due to introduction of the vaccine several years ago. **Research is indicating that people who have been vaccinated are less likely to experience shingles than those who had the disease.** One dose of chicken pox vaccine is given at age 1 year. If children are over the age of 13 when they are vaccinated, they must have two doses.

In all, eleven dangerous infections can be prevented through routine childhood immunization. All childhood vaccines have undergone years of study to refine them and decrease associated risk. Today's vaccines are very safe, usually causing only low grade fever, soreness at the injection site, and fussiness as side effects. Severe reactions to vaccines are *extremely rare*. The benefits of vaccines *far* outweigh the risks. Historically some of these diseases caused epidemics leading to thousands of deaths. How wonderful it is to have the opportunity to provide this protection for your child!

WELL CHILD CARE

Dr. Paul Antal is convinced that "the best step to prevent health problems in your child is regular visits to your health care provider."

Prenatal care comes first as discussed in Chapter 1. Then, in the newborn period, your baby will have several complete examinations to rule out any birth defects or problems with adjustment to life outside the womb. Up to 5% of newborns have some abnormality, so it's essential that they are evaluated to identify and treat any problems.

After the newborn period, the American Academy of Pediatrics recommends a schedule of well child visits — your heath care provider will discuss this with you. These check-ups are *essential* as physical and developmental problems can occur at any time, and the sooner they are identified, the sooner they can be taken care of. In addition, immunizations are usually given at these visits. After the age of 2, checkups are usually yearly. Often parents think that once their child has started school they only need to visit their health care provider when they are sick — *not true!* There are many issues and problems which must be screened for as your child grows and becomes a teenager. These are easy exams and can save a lot of heartache by providing prevention rather than a catchup attempt at intervention after the fact. In addition, it's wonderful to see how well your child is growing and thriving at their check ups!

Dental care is also important. Tooth brushing should be started as soon as your child has several teeth. Fluoride supplements are recommended if your water supply is not fluoridated — this helps prevent cavity formation. Visits to the dentist should begin in the toddler or preschool period, whichever your dentist prefers.

HAND WASHING

Routine as it may seem, one of the best disease prevention tools is hand washing, according to Dr. Pamela Bradt.

Most communicable diseases are transmitted either by dirty hands or by coughing and sneezing. Hand washing will prevent many of these. Bacteria and viruses seem to be trapped by the skin oils all of us have. Soap, plain or fancy, acts by lifting the skin oils off and floating them away. On top of this, many bacteria have cell walls with lots of fat in them so the soaps damage the cell walls in addition to washing them away. Wash your hands regularly. Do so every time you go to the bathroom, every time you sneeze if you have a cold, every time you handle your pets, and every time you change your baby's diaper. All this seems obvious, but watch how many people use public restrooms and do not stop at the sink on the way out. And watch how many stop at the sink, but don't use soap. **We are our own worst enemies.**

Do wash your hands, but don't use an antibacterial soap. They aren't necessary unless you have an immune deficiency which may accompany cancer, AIDS or something similar. The vast majority of us do not need the antibacterial or antibiotic soaps. In fact, we do more harm when we use them. Bacteria don't like being attacked and look for ways around every new antibiotic, developing resistance. Each time we use antibacterial soaps unnecessarily, we help those bacteria on the road to developing resistance. Soon they will not be destroyed by soap. This is especially true in hospitals where antibiotics and antibacterial soaps are necessary. Let's not make our homes like hospitals.

DON'T SHARE YOUR GERMS

It seems like common sense, but cover your mouth, and teach your children to, each time you or they sneeze or cough — then wash your hands. These two easy motions can significantly reduce the spread of respiratory illness. Many preschools are now teaching children to sneeze into the crook of their arm if they will be unable to wash their hands immediately.

Dr. Sheldon Korones goes as far as to suggest that new babies be kissed on the top of the head to avoid transmission of respiratory infection.

Infants are particularly vulnerable to infection, so extra care should be taken. Avoiding kissing babies on their mouths has been shown in studies to reduce the incidence of dental decay in children. Adults and older children with cold sores should avoid direct contact with infants as many cold sores are caused by the herpes virus which can cause meningitis in infants.

Avoid Overuse of Antibiotics

*Dr. David McNeeley warns: "Antibiotics
have no role in the treatment of the
common cold and overuse of them
promotes the development of resistant
bacteria."*

This is so true! Don't ask for or take antibiotics for upper respiratory infections. They are all caused by viruses which are not susceptible to antibiotics. All you do is help more bacteria become resistant to antibiotics with no improvement in your cold. If you or your child have a throat infection, your health care provider can do a throat culture which will show if it is viral or bacterial in origin. If viral, antibiotics are not necessary and should not be given. If streptococcal (bacterial), antibiotics are needed, but only then.

If you or your child do have antibiotics prescribed for a bacterial infection, take all of the medication given to you. Stopping early because you feel better may lead to a recurrence of the infection or may lead to your bacteria becoming resistant because you didn't eradicate it completely. Finish taking all of the antibiotics prescribed for you. Do not take antibiotics someone else has left over. First of all, you probably don't need them. Second, you don't know it's the correct one for you. Third, you won't have enough to do the job. Fourth, your health care provider won't know. And fifth, both your friend and you are helping bacteria to develop resistance!

The old adage, 'an ounce of prevention is worth a pound of cure' is so applicable to the care of our children. As parents, it's best to be armed with all the information possible to safe guard your children's health — your health care provider can guide you through the process, *if* you see them regularly!

CHECKLIST

Use this Checklist to track your progress in meeting the recommendations in this chapter.

Goal	Accomplished		Will do		By When Date
	Yes	No	Yes	No	
Immunize your child with DTaP — Diphtheria, Tetanus and Pertussis					
Immunize for polio					
Immunize for Hib — Hemophilus Influenza Type B					
Immunize for Hep B — Hepatitis B					
Immunize for Pneumococcus					
Immunize for MMR — Measles, Mumps and Rubella					
Immunize for Chicken Pox					
Make and keep all recommended well baby and child care appointments					
Teach your child to brush their teeth					
Use fluoride					
See the dentist					
Wash your hands and teach your children to do so					
No antibacterial soap unless prescribed					
Cover mouth when coughing and sneezing					
Do not take antibiotics for colds					
If prescribed, take all the antibiotic					
Do not take someone else's medicine					

Chapter 3
Make Home a Safe Haven

YOUR HOME SHOULD BE A SANCTUARY for your family. While it is impossible to make it completely safe, there are many ways to reduce the risks for your children. Parents tend to be more relaxed at home and not as observant of potential dangers as when they are in public places. Keep in mind, the majority of accidents happen to children in or near their homes. Beginning with infancy, here are some suggestions to consider to make your home a truly safe haven for your child.

BACK LYING SLEEP POSITION

> *Dr. Sheldon Korones strongly advocates that "After your baby is born, and until he or she can roll over on their own, always place them on their back."*

There seems to be little argument that the incidence of sudden infant death syndrome is higher if infants are placed on their sides or stomach to sleep. It's probably related to exhaled carbon dioxide accumulating in the bedding and thereby effectively lowering the available oxygen leading to an abnormal heart rhythm and sudden death.

CHOOSE A SAFE CRIB

Your baby's crib should be approved by the Consumer Product Safety Commission (CPSC). Its rungs should be close enough together to prevent your fist from going between them. While the crib you slept in as a child may have a lot of sentimental value, it is not a safe choice for your baby today. Many injuries, and even deaths, have occurred when infant's heads become wedged between the bars of unsafe cribs. Don't use bumper pads in your baby's crib. They look pretty, but babies can smother in them when their faces become stuck against them. When a child is older and more mobile, they can use bumper pads to help in climbing over the side of the crib, which can lead to injury. The same is true for pillows and stuffed toys. Babies can smother with them.

MAKE YOUR CHILD'S SURROUNDINGS SAFE

As your child becomes more mobile and independent (around six months of age) you will need to look at your home in a different light. Your baby will be spending more time on the floor and many more dangers will present themselves. Get down on your floor and crawl around as your baby does and look at the things in your path. Simple household items may pose a threat to small children. Examples include:

- **Potted Plants** — Your child may ingest the leaves or dirt.
- **Pet Foods** -They are potential choking hazards and, while not poisonous, they contain substances not meant for humans.
- **Corners** — Furniture, counter tops, and fireplaces may cause injury to small heads which come up underneath them as they stand or fall against them. Corner guards are readily available in stores for your counters. Throw a quilt on your hearth and your coffee table until your child is a steady walker.
- **Electrical Outlets** — Outlets and cords are fascinating to young children. Electrocution or severe burns can occur from sticking an object into an electrical outlet or from chewing on an electrical cord. Dr. Karla Smith's first safety recommendation is to cover outlets with CPSC approved covers — readily available in stores. Put electrical cords underneath heavy furniture or up high where they are not accessible to small hands and mouths.
- **Glass Fireplace Doors** — they are a magnet for small children who press their noses and palms against the glass to see the pretty light. Burns may result. A fireplace screen won't keep your baby from crawling into or too close to the fire. If you have a fire you must stay within arms length of your baby or toddler at all times.
- **Child Safety Locks** — When your baby starts crawling, you will need to put child locks on all your under counter cabinets and on many closets and bifold doors. Children are very curious and will pull open cabinet doors as they explore. Anything in-

side is fair game — garbage, cleaning fluids, dishes, pots and pans, food or whatever. Everything they find will go into their mouths since that's their best developed sensory organ at that age.

- **Child Gates** — Place a child gate at the top and bottom of all stairs. Little crawlers can go up or down anything, sometimes very quickly. A tumble down the stairs will ruin everyone's day. If the gate is made of wood with rungs, be sure they are too close together to prevent your fist from going through. Also, if you have a banister with spindles, they should not allow an adult fist between them or else a child's head can become wedged as well.

- **Lock All Doors and Windows** — If necessary put a chain or slide lock up high at the top of doors. If a child decides to explore the outdoors or the garage while you're asleep, the results could be devastating. Falls from windows can be just as disastrous. Don't count on a screen to stop your child from falling. If you have double hung windows, open them from the top. Take cranks off or use child safe cranks (available from the window manufacturer).

- **Always Supervise Your Children** — Most accidents happen when parents turn their backs for only a few minutes. Don't count on the buckle strap in a high chair to restrain your child. They are amazing climbers. Put your infant in their crib, a playpen or a port-a-crib when you need to turn your attention elsewhere, such as to take a shower.

Dr. Ward Griffen warns: "Parents truly do need to have eyes in the backs of their heads."

Poisons

Put all your cleaning agents and medications up high. Probably the best is a high cabinet in the kitchen, bathroom or laundry room. Ideally, you should have a lock and key on those cabinets until your children are old enough to understand the danger. Something that seems as innocuous as baby oil and other household products containing hydrocarbons, when swallowed by children, get thrown up and aspirated into the lungs, possibly causing a chemical pneumonia. As of October 2002, such products will have to be sold in child-resistant packaging.

Keep all bath, body and massage oils, sunscreens and makeup removers well away from small children. Handle medicines seriously and teach your children to respect them. Never refer to any medicine as 'candy.' In spite of this your children may get into something they shouldn't. It's a good idea to have some syrup of ipecac in the house to make them vomit when they swallow something that they shouldn't. In addition, keep the number of your closest Poison Control Center beside all telephones. **NEVER administer ipecac before first calling Poison Control. Inducing vomiting may worsen the injury from some poisons.**

Baby Walkers

Don't use baby walkers! The temptation to put your baby in one of them is great. They're so much fun to watch — but, don't use them. First of all, children can get away from you much too quickly. Most importantly, your baby needs to learn to crawl and then to pull up and walk the old fashioned way. Time spent in walkers is associated with delayed walking and persistent toe walking. Falls down stairs in walkers can cause severe head injuries. In addition, walkers elevate your child and make them able to reach items placed on tables, counters and stoves, presenting more dangers.

Kitchen Safety

As your children grow, they will want to be with you, especially in the kitchen. Teach them about hot things so that they stay away from them. Make sure they never try to open the oven.

Dr. Margaret Griffen tells parents to always turn pot and sauce pan handles away from the edge of the stove.

They are too great a temptation. Glass oven doors get very hot and can cause burns when children touch or attempt to look through them. Make sure all knives, scissors, sharp tools and objects are in a locked drawer or up high. Keep in mind that as soon as they are able to climb, your children will pull chairs over to counters and climb up on them. The same is true in the garage. Saws, axes and other tools are magnets for children.

Bath Tub Safety

Always stay beside the tub or sink when bathing your baby or young child. You really must be within arms reach at all times. This means you should have everything you'll need ready at hand before you begin. It also means you cannot answer the telephone and give a bath at the same time. Using a cordless or wireless phone, or a phone with a long cord isn't a good idea either. **All your attention should be focused on your baby throughout the bath.** If you have other children, they must be accounted for so that you aren't distracted. Bathing your baby during nap time for the others works well. If they are older perhaps they can be entertained by helping during the bath. Remember, a baby can get in real trouble in just seconds. Once his or her face is under water and water is inhaled, everything shuts down to keep the water out of the lungs. An abnormal heart rhythm can occur very quickly with disastrous results. Other water sources are a risk for young children. Drain water from all sinks and tubs immediately — a child can fall in and drown. Don't soak your dishes in a full sink or leave your mop bucket full. **Close the lid on toilets.**

CHOKING

Keep small items out of reach. Check all your child's toys to be sure there are no removable parts or that the toy itself is so small that they may be swallowed. If they can be, your baby can choke on the toy. The best is to not have such toys around. Remember other items in your home may be choking hazards or may be put into noses or ears, such as marbles, paper clips, or erasers to mention a few.

Dr. Karla Smith is especially emphatic about avoiding foods which can cause choking.

Don't feed your child popcorn, nuts, raw carrots, hot dogs, hard candy, chewing gum or similar foods until they are three years or older. Also make sure they don't help themselves to such foods you are eating.

FIREARMS

Lock All Firearms or Decide Not To Have Them in Your Home — **ALL** firearms should be locked in a gun safe or closet. They should always be unloaded and the ammunition should be stored in a separate locked place. The keys should be kept in a third secure place. Children are curious and do not comprehend the dangers guns pose. They may think a gun is a toy or may mimic behavior they have seen on TV.

We firmly believe that loaded guns, unsecured, are a disaster waiting to happen.

Emergency Measures

Have a Fire Safety Plan. You should have a plan in place to evacuate your house or apartment in the event of a fire. Know how to get to your child and how to get out safely. As your children grow, they must be taught how to evacuate alone, down the fire escape or out the window. Have a rope ladder or whatever is necessary to provide for their safety. Practice your plan at least twice a year at the daylight savings time change. When your children are older, designate a specific meeting place for your family outside your home. Remember to have working smoke detectors in your home and to change the batteries twice a year, also at the daylight savings time change.

Know the Heimlich Maneuver and CPR and teach your children when they are old enough. CPR classes (which include treatment of choking) are readily available through your local hospital, often as part of childbirth and parenting classes, through the Red Cross or the American Heart Association. Make sure to take a course which includes infants and children when you have young children in your home.

Finally, teach your children to use the telephone to dial 911 or the appropriate number in your area. You may not always be around or something may happen to you so that they need to call for help. This lesson may save your life as well as your child's.

Implementing these suggestions in your home will help you create the safe haven you want.

CHECKLIST

Use this Checklist to track your progress in meeting the recommendations in this chapter.

Goal	Accomplished		Will do		By When
	Yes	No	Yes	No	Date
Place your baby to sleep on his or her back					
Use a safe crib					
No bumper pads, pillows or toys in the crib					
Potted plants placed up high or outside					
Pet foods never left out					
Corners are rounded or covered					
Cover all electrical outlets					
Put electrical cords under rugs, furniture or up high					
Watch glass fireplace doors					
Use child safety locks on doors and cabinets					
Lock up cleaning agents and medicines					
Post Poison Control Center number near all phones					
Have syrup of ipecac on hand, use under direction only					
Use child gates					
Check space between banister spindles					
Don't use baby walkers					
Use kitchen safety — sharps, handles and hot oven or stove					
Use garage safety — tools, dangerous liquids, cars, etc.					
Never leave a child unattended in the bath tub					
Lock doors and windows					
Always supervise your child					
No firearms in house or keep locked					
Have fire safety plan					
Know CPR and Heimlich Maneuver					
Teach your child how to call 911					

Chapter 4
The World Can Be a Scary Place

WHEN YOU LEAVE YOUR HOME you have less control over all the possible threats to your child's safety. It's hard to anticipate every risk, but there are many we can significantly reduce by using common sense and following approved safety recommendations.

SEAT BELTS AND CAR SEATS

All states have child restraint laws. Some states are more strict that others. Many also have seat belt laws.

- All states require that infants below 20 lbs or one year of age, whichever comes first, ride in an approved rear facing infant car seat in the back seat of your vehicle. Infant car seats are available to rent or borrow from most hospitals. The slogan "Make your baby's first ride a safe ride" is really true. Holding your child in your arms in a moving vehicle is never a safe option. The death and severe injury rate for children has dropped dramatically since child safety seats have been required.

- When your baby is 20 lbs or one year of age you may move them to a front facing safety seat in the back seat of the vehicle. Depending on the type of safety seat you have, your child should stay in it until they are 40 to 60 lbs. Then they should move to a booster seat until 80 lbs or when they are tall enough for the shoulder seat belt to fit across their hips rather than their abdomen (at about 8 years of age). Again, your child should always be in the back seat. It is the safest place in the vehicle.
- A recent study showed that riders with an automatic shoulder belt but manual lap belt didn't fasten the lap belt 50 to 70% of the time. Researchers found that not using the lap belt carries a higher risk for chest and abdominal injuries than using no belt at all. Make sure that everyone has fastened his or her lap belt before you start the car.
- Seat belts have been proven to reduce serious injury and deaths. Be a good role model: protect yourself by wearing your seat belt at all times.

HELMETS

Another important life saving device is the helmet.

Dr. Ward Griffen urges that an approved helmet be worn while biking, rollerblading, scootering or skateboarding.

Ice skating, skiing, snow boarding, and horseback riding also necessitate helmet use. Many competitive and team sports require helmets (i.e. football and ice hockey). Helmets are made specifically for each of these individual sports. A bicycle helmet approved by ANSI (American National Standards Institute) or the Snell Foundation can cover biking and all the roller sports. All other sports require helmets made specifically for that sport for the best protection. The incidence of head injuries has significantly declined since sports safety helmets were introduced.

- Helmets are absolutely necessary and required by law in most states on motorized vehicles such as motorcycles, all terrain vehicles and snowmobiles.

WATER SAFETY

Water is a wonderful place for recreation and exercise; but it can be deadly without proper safety precautions. Drowning is a leading cause of death from accidental injury in children and it's virtually 100% preventable! The key to prevention of water accidents is *adult supervision.*

> *Dr. Margaret Griffen wants parents to know how to swim themselves and then enroll their children in swimming lessons if they are available.*

Begin when they are toddlers and continue until they are accomplished independent swimmers. All children should wear life jackets *in* and *around* the water until they are independent swimmers. Life jackets must also be worn in any water craft (this is law in most states) at all times. Remember, the key again is attentive adult supervision.

- Use sunscreen when you are outdoors, even if it's not hot. Sun exposure in all races and skin types is cumulative beginning at birth. Tans look great, but without sunscreen they lead to skin cancer, the most common form of cancer.
- Use at least SPF 15 in children over 6 months and for yourself. For infants under 6 months, keep them in the shade and cover their skin with light clothing and a sun hat.
- In addition to skin cancer, sun exposure causes wrinkles and aging of the skin. If good skin habits are started in childhood they will become lifelong.
- Remember to give liquids frequently while outdoors if it is hot.
- In public swimming pools, beware of swallowing too much water. It may contain bacteria or parasites which can cause severe gastrointestinal distress — diarrhea and nausea — as well as fever several days after swallowing the contaminated water.

ANIMAL SAFETY

Safety around animals is often overlooked and can lead to tragic results. The natural reaction for most children is curiosity and the desire to touch and get close to animals, especially dogs and cats. Encourage this curiosity from a distance. Teach your children to be cautious around animals and explain that some are not friendly. Be sure the animal is controlled or leashed and ask the owner's permission before going near. If you don't know the owner, it's probably best to stay away. Dog bites can be deadly and horribly disfiguring, and all animal bites or scratches are potential sources of infection.

- Use caution when choosing a pet for your family. Some breeds of dogs are not meant to be pets. Know the background or previous owners of any pet before bringing it into your home. Obtain appropriate veterinary care for the animal before exposing your children to it.
- Be aware that your children may experience allergic reactions to animals. It may be useful to visit with another family's pet(s) before making a decision about a pet for your family.
- Wild animals are meant to be in the wild. They should be observed from afar and not approached *ever.*
- If your child is bitten or severely scratched by a wild or domestic animal, call your health care provider immediately about rabies prevention.

STRANGER SAFETY

Talk with your children about strangers. Never leave your child with someone you don't know **well**. Your child needs to consider any adult or older child, whom they don't know, as a stranger until you tell them otherwise. Teach your child the correct way to answer the door and telephone in your home when they are old enough. Explain what to do if a stranger approaches them — walk or run away and tell an adult they trust.

- Knowledge can be a lifesaver for your child. Before he or she starts kindergarten, practice your address, phone number, city and state with them. It can be a game you play each time you get into the car. Make sure your child knows each parent's first and last name (it may be different from their own) and their workplaces.
- Make sure your child knows how to contact you or another specified adult in an emergency, i.e., if they need a ride, are in an unsafe situation, or simply if they come home to an empty house because you're late.

GUN SAFETY

Firearms are made with the intent to cause serious injury or to kill. Carefully consider the choice of having them in your home. If you do decide to have firearms, remember the safety guidelines discussed in chapter 3. Anticipate the possibility of your child coming into contact with firearms in some one else's home or outdoors, in the garage, etc. Teach them that all objects which look like guns must be treated as guns until a trusted adult says otherwise. They should never touch a gun, but should notify an adult immediately. If a playmate touches a gun they should *run away* and tell the adult in charge. Guns in the hands of children lead to nothing but heartbreak.

The world can indeed be a scary place. It will help to know that you've done all you can to make it safer for your children. Since many things are beyond our control, make sure to take every step possible to prevent tragedy from striking.

CHECKLIST

Use this Checklist to track your progress in meeting the recommendations in this chapter.

Goal	Accomplished Yes	No	Will do Yes	No	By When Date
Use child safety seats					
Children belong in the back seat					
Use seat belts					
Use appropriate helmets					
Wear life jackets around water					
Learn to swim and teach your child					
Use sun screen					
Cover infants under six months in the sun					
Use caution around animals					
Choose pets wisely					
Teach appropriate behavior around strangers					
Teach proper door and telephone answering					
Teach your address, city, state and telephone number					
Teach your and your mate's first and last name and work place					
Leave emergency contact numbers					
Secure or remove all guns from home					
Teach gun safety					

Chapter 5
You've Only Got One Body

EACH OF US HAS ONLY ONE BODY in which to live our lives, so why poison it with harmful substances?

DON'T BE AN ASHTRAY

- Exposure to cigarette smoke in their homes is a terrible health threat for children. Exposure to smoke contributes to higher rates of Sudden Infant Death Syndrome, chronic lung disease such as asthma, more frequent upper respiratory infections and ear infections, and an increased risk of allergies.
- Researchers have found that just a small amount of secondhand smoke can cause measurable damage to a child's learning ability, affecting reading, math and reasoning.
- Babies whose mothers smoke during pregnancy have a higher rate of prematurity and lower birth weight even when full term.

When you make the choice to become parents, make the choice to make your home smoke free. This means smoke *outside* or stop smoking. Going to another room or standing by an exhaust fan is inadequate. Smoking only when your children are not home is also not acceptable since the tar is deposited on your walls, draperies, upholstery and clothing. Smoking in your car creates the same problem, even if you only smoke in it when your children are not present. If you are unable to stop smoking, do so only outdoors and wear a jacket which you remove prior to coming in to protect your clothing. If you hold your infant against smoky clothing, they still inhale tar.

• Don't allow visitors in your home to smoke.

Children learn what they see. Don't be a role model for smoking (cigarettes, cigars, pipes) or the use of smokeless tobacco (snuff, chewing tobacco) for your children. Smoking has been proven to cause lung cancer and to be associated with many other forms of cancer. Smokeless tobacco causes mouth, tongue and throat cancer. You'll shorten your life and your children's lives by smoking and teaching them to smoke. Talk about smoking with your children and help them understand the health risks and how unattractive it is. Anti-smoking campaigns in schools are very comprehensive, but **learning about the dangers of smoking should begin well before your child starts school.** Smoking is more common in movies again, so be observant. Support campaigns to rate movies on smoking as well as language, violence and sex. Beliefs and opinions are established early. Don't be a 'do as I say, not as I do' parent. Don't smoke or quit.

If your older child comes home smelling like smoke, take it seriously, says Dr. Stephen Dilts.

- Don't accept your child's explanation that they were around someone else who was smoking. Intervene and set limits.
- Cigarettes cannot legally be sold in most states to children under age eighteen, but don't assume this will restrict your child's access to cigarettes.

DRINKING ALCOHOL

CAN BE DANGEROUS

Alcohol is a legal substance if you meet the age requirement in your state. However, drinking and driving is never legal or safe, and drinking while pregnant is always harmful. It is important to present a clear message to your children about the appropriate use of alcohol. Research has shown that alcohol in moderation (one or two drinks a day) may help prevent heart disease. The key is moderation. Alcohol in chronic excess can cause liver, stomach and brain damage. Most importantly, alcohol impairs judgment and reflexes. Be a role model for responsible use of alcohol and only for adults. Alcohol is never appropriate for children or teenagers.

- Alcohol is the cause of large numbers of teen auto accidents along with boating and drowning accidents.
- Judgment is impaired when a young person uses alcohol. They may make a choice to use drugs or have sex that they might otherwise not have made.

Illegal Drugs Are Lethal

Drug use is illegal and dangerous in every form and for everyone. Remember children are observant and learn and do what they see. Don't use drugs or allow them in your home. Talk to your children about their dangers.

- Drugs may actually be more available to your children than alcohol or tobacco because drugs are sold or shared on the street, at school or at parties. They are not sold in stores.
- Many inhalants are available in your home in the form of model glue or aerosol cans for whipped cream, cleaning agents and hair spray.

Dr. Stephen Dilts believes a parent's top priority is to pay attention to the choices their children may be making.

Pay attention to your children. Sudden or gradual changes in appearance, behavior or habits, dropping grades or poor school attendance, and different friends may all be signs of drug or alcohol abuse. Drugs and alcohol can destroy lives!

CHECKLIST

Use this Checklist to track your progress in meeting the recommendations in this chapter.

Goal	Accomplished		Will do		By When
	Yes	No	Yes	No	Date
No smoking					
Check out evidence of smoking in older children					
Limit your own alcohol use					
Never drink and drive					
Don't mix alcohol with boating					
Never use illegal drugs					
Be aware of inhalants					
Pay attention to older children's behavior					
Remember you are a role model whether you think you are or not					

Chapter 6
Put Family First

As soon as you bring your newborn home you begin the lifelong process of being a family — father, mother, brothers and/or sisters.

FAMILY TIME

Make family time a priority. Take walks together, visit relatives and friends together, and try to arrange schedules so that you can have breakfast and supper together. By doing this you create the opportunity for family discussions as your children grow and ask questions, and, above all, you keep in touch with each other.

- Family vacations are a great way to spend time together away from all the demands of jobs and home. Long weekends or one or two weeks vacation at the beach or some other place fun for all are the best idea. If that doesn't work, a couple of days at home with no commitments will suffice.
- Schedule one night a week that is set aside for family time. Call it family game or family movie night. Plan something fun. Take turns deciding what you will do together.

SELF ESTEEM

AND MENTAL HEALTH

As your children grow, remember that discipline must be sweetened by positive reinforcement. Praise what they learn to do well and creatively suggest improvement in things done a little less well than desired. Make reading, drawing, coloring, cutting and pasting fun. Display their creations on the refrigerator or doors or walls. You should keep some of these in your treasure chest. They're fun to look at, especially if and when your children have children of their own, who would love to see their parent's childhood artwork.

Dr. Matthew Boulis recommends:
"Be sure to positively reinforce your children from infancy to young adulthood in a manner that will help them develop a strong sense of self worth and a confident image. There is no better armament to face the trials of the real world."

Children face so many obstacles as they grow and learn, the one place they must feel unconditional acceptance is at home. Make sure your child or teen knows that, while you may not always like their behavior, you will always love them. Don't push them to only succeed, but to put forth their best effort. Point out their strengths and encourage growth in areas of weakness — **never belittle.**

- Mental illness in children is reaching epidemic proportions. Be alert to your child's feelings and behavior. Don't overlook 'down' type behavior in young children. If they avoid school or friends, or withdraw in other ways, seek professional help. **Be available and be observant.**

Many young teenagers have problems with depression and associated anxiety or panic. Some probably is normal in all young people. But depression which leads to slovenly dress, poor eating habits or over eating, dramatic mood swings, unkempt hair and body, and any other warning signs must be taken seriously. Professional counseling is a must. You as the parent cannot count on your child's school catching the problem or fixing it. Most of the time, however, they will be helpful and may even alert you to the problem. Don't depend on them — pay attention and take appropriate action. It's *your* responsibility. It's *your* child!

PRIVACY AND HONESTY

Putting family first also demands respect for privacy. As covered in chapter 9, bathrooms are private if the door is closed. If your child has a private room, it should be just that — private. You as a parent have the duty to be sure it is clean and neat, that toys are put away and that clothes are properly stored and laundry taken out. You also have the duty to notice if other activities are taking place which shouldn't, such as smoking. Privacy extends both directions. Loud music from behind a closed door may be very irritating to others in the family. It invades their privacy. Earphones are one solution, but the best is music at a reasonable level protecting the ears of all around. Remember, a family shares a home and each member's needs are important.

Answer your child's questions honestly. Do not be afraid to say "I don't know." Deferring answers to your mate indicates you are uncomfortable discussing it yourself. You may say "Mom and Dad need to talk this over first to decide the best way to answer you." Don't stoop to the archaic copout, "Wait 'til your father gets home." Confront your child's questions, don't avoid them. If you give the message, even with your body language, that you don't want to talk about something, your child will seek answers elsewhere. Other sources may not answer within your family's moral framework.

> *Dr. Boulis says flatly, "Never lie to your child, Be honest and explain why you can or can't meet their demands. Remember all children have 'needs and wants' and you as a parent have to fulfill their needs but not all of their wants. This will help them mature."*

If you expect honesty from your children you will have to be honest with them. Sometimes they won't need all the details or rationale — just "Mom and Dad think this is the best choice." Don't beat around the bush or tell partial truths unless you want to be answered that way by your child — *remember one way or another, you will be the most important role model in their lives.*

VIOLENCE

Home is the first and best place to teach appropriate conflict resolution. It doesn't matter how many programs a child attends in school — the methods he learns at home are the ones that stick.

- Set a positive example as much as you can. Keep arguments between you and your mate at a minimum and behind closed doors, if possible. Healthy discussion is fine; children need to learn how to talk out problems.

Beginning with a toddler who bites another child who takes their toy, it is important to recognize that violence between children happens. Usually it can be avoided by paying attention and controlling the situation before things reach that stage. Especially for boys, learning how to settle quarrels without resorting to physical aggression is part of growing up. Teach them to say "I'm sorry" without fear and to try to reason through a problem first. Encourage using their words rather than their bodies to express anger. Try to get them to count to ten before reacting to avoid outbursts — this applies to parents also!

TALKING ABOUT SEX

Learning about sex is a very important piece of a child's maturation. Your role as a parent is to help them through the process of questioning and understanding. Many things are explained in school health curricula, but the primary responsibility lies with you, the parent.

> *Cathy Carter asks: "Do you really want*
> *your child to learn about sex from a*
> *stranger in a classroom full of other*
> *children, or worse, on the school bus*
> *from another child?"*

Take the opportunity to educate your child according to your family's morals. Once they have heard it else-where, you lose the chance to present the information in the way you would choose for the first time. First impressions are very important.

With all the sexuality expressed in the media, you may be questioned by your young children. Be frank, and don't offer more than what they've asked. Older children will eventually want to know where babies come from. Usually, at first, that means how do they get out of your stomach, not anything more. Be simple and explain more if they aren't satisfied. Be prepared to explain reproduction in general terms. Obviously, avoid inappropriate language or slang terms. It's better to use the proper names of the parts and organs involved. If your child feels it necessary to use those terms in the wrong place, you can deal with that at the time.

- Sex is a natural part of our lives. For those who live near rural areas, seeing animals mating or giving birth is to be expected and can be used to begin the explanation of where babies come from. Don't avoid it. If you do your children will learn from older children who will generally get it wrong or make it sound other than what it is — a natural and loving part of an adult relationship.

While this may be a difficult and sensitive part of your job as a parent — everyone has different comfort levels with regard to sex — it nevertheless *is* one of the most important things you'll do!

GOALS

Remember the saying,
"If you don't know where you're going,
any road will get you there."

Your children should know your goals in life and you should discuss with them their own goals for their lives. At first, until 6th grade or so, goals should be a matter of demonstration or role modeling. They learn best by mimicking you. You should not drive them to achievement rather than insisting that they do their best. Driven children sooner or later jump off the wagon and the fall can be very hard. In middle or junior high school, they do need to begin some goal choices. Grades become more and more important and finding areas of interest which might indicate future career direction must be taken seriously.

By high school, the need for goals is even more critical. If you intend for your child to go to college, and he or she wants to, the correct curriculum must be chosen and grades become very important. College and university choices don't need to be made until junior year, but clearly study up to that point must be directed toward that opportunity. If your child wants a technical career instead, the appropriate curriculum should be chosen. In all of this, remember *it's the goal of your child, not necessarily yours, which is important.*

SPIRITUALITY

Talk with your children about spirituality beginning in their early years. We recommend all families involve themselves in the spiritual life of their chosen belief. All will have programs for youth which provide useful peer support in a safe and wholesome atmosphere. Having strong spiritual beliefs can fill the void, especially for teenagers, when they are searching for their place in life. With so many unknowns, and so many obstacles to face as they become adults, having faith to rely on can be a great source of strength. Family is the main avenue for exposure to spirituality for children. Make sure to share your beliefs with your children and involve them in organized worship.

Historically, the family was the source of all socialization and education — anything known was learned at home. Today children face a multitude of outside influences — **it's time for parents to reclaim and take responsibility for those issues which should *first* be taught at home.**

CHECKLIST

Use this Checklist to track your progress in meeting the recommendations in this chapter.

Goal	Accomplished Yes	No	Will do Yes	No	By When Date
Have fun together as a family					
Try to take family vacations					
Eat meals together					
Praise your children when they do well					
Be gentle with correction					
Never belittle your children					
Pay attention to behavior changes, especially in teens					
Seek professional counseling when appropriate					
Respect privacy					
Answer questions honestly					
Be a positive role model concerning violence					
Discuss sex before others do					
Discuss life goals					
Encourage spiritual life as important and helpful					

Chapter 7
You Really Are What You Eat

GOOD NUTRITION BEGINS in the prenatal period as discussed in chapter 1. Food is fuel for your body and nutritious foods maximize your child's growth and development. Healthy eating habits begin in infancy and can really contribute to your child's overall health throughout their life.

INFANT FEEDING

After your baby is born, optimally you will breast feed exclusively for the first several months. After other foods are added, breastfeeding is recommended in addition until at least one year of age.

- While you are nursing, keep up your own well balanced nutritious diet, remembering you need around 900 *extra* calories a day to maintain high quality breast milk. You can cut these calories in half to 450 in order to lose weight, if that's a problem. You shouldn't go lower.
- Remember to avoid caffeine and especially alcohol and drugs, while you are nursing. They are passed to your baby through your milk.

- Take only medicines prescribed by your health care provider.
- Don't smoke while you are breastfeeding. Nicotine is passed through your breast milk.

If you are unable to breast feed or if it is your choice not to, your baby should be given iron fortified infant formula until one year of age. Occasionally your health care provider will approve a change to cow's milk sooner, but don't do this on your own. The formula you choose may be milk based or soy based depending on what your baby tolerates. Your health care provider will help you with this choice.

It is imperative that you give full iron formula to your baby if you are not breastfeeding to prevent iron deficiency anemia. It is a misconception that iron in formula causes constipation in babies. Scientific studies have shown that, at most, iron in formula causes darker colored stools.

Dr. Pamela Bradt emphasizes that,
"if your formula fed baby is truly
constipated with hard pellet-like stools
and going three to four days between
stools, you should talk to your health
care provider about ways to help this."

Do not give low iron formula.

Solid Foods

It is best to wait until four to six months of age to introduce solid foods such as cereal and baby foods. Earlier introduction of foods other than breast milk or formula may lead to a higher incidence of food allergy and malabsorption disorders.

> *Dr. Allan Weingold stresses that*
> *"you pay attention to any*
> *family history of allergies."*

You'll get lots of advice from family members on this issue: "You ate cereal when you were two weeks old," etc. Rely on your health care provider to guide you with the addition of solid foods.

Feeding Your Toddler

There will be times when you will wonder how your toddler gains any weight at all! One of your basic instincts as a parent is to *feed your child* and this instinct will be challenged repeatedly in the toddler and preschool period. Infants who were wonderful, well balanced eaters may turn into toddlers who eat a repertoire of three or four things and love a food one day and detest it the next. This is all very normal developmentally and is referred to as 'food jags' in toddlers and preschoolers — frustration time for the parents!

It doesn't matter that your child eats the same things all the time, but it is important that they are nutritious and represent all the food groups.

Dr. Karen Funk recommends that you use the food pyramid as your guide for healthy eating. See below to refresh your memory.

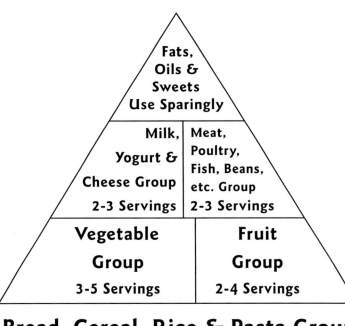

Fats, Oils & Sweets
Use Sparingly

Milk, Yogurt & Cheese Group
2-3 Servings

Meat, Poultry, Fish, Beans, etc. Group
2-3 Servings

Vegetable Group
3-5 Servings

Fruit Group
2-4 Servings

Bread, Cereal, Rice & Pasta Group
6-11 Servings

Make sure your child is eating nutritiously over time. Look at the week as a whole rather than one day at a time and your child's food intake may actually be better than you think. Don't give in and let your child eat junk because you are afraid they will starve. If they are hungry enough they will eat. Offer a variety of healthy foods and let your toddler make choices. Dessert foods are *never* necessary and should be reserved as occasional 'treats.'

Establish regular mealtimes with the family in the toddler period. While your child may not be able to sit through the entire meal, they should learn the mealtime routine and sit with you to eat. A regular mealtime is a very important part of family life and should be established early. Turn off the TV and sit down at the table together for as many meals as possible for your family's schedule.

- Establish a 'no grazing' rule. If you let your toddler snack constantly or walk around with a sipper cup or bottle (these should be gone *before* 18 months), they never feel hungry and won't eat at mealtime.
- Schedule six small feedings a day — three regular meals and three healthy snacks — not sugary foods. Have your child sit at the table each time they eat.
- While it's difficult, if you are serving good food, your older children should eat what is placed in front of them. It may be a little challenging at first, but they will learn to expand their eating horizons with time. Be sure to set a good example.
- Refuse to be a short order cook. It's an impossible habit to break! Everyone has preferences, but children should be willing to try new things.

Beverages

Choose healthy beverages for your child — remember they are foods, too. Children should drink whole cow's milk until at least age 2 unless you are directed otherwise by your health care provider. They need the milk fat to stimulate brain growth. After age 2 switch to 2% milk or less depending on what your family drinks. Milk and dairy products are very important for your child's bone growth. Calcium is absorbed best from dairy products. Four servings a day will meet this requirement. Calcium is especially important for adolescents who are manufacturing bone mass. They need 1000 mg of calcium a day to maximize bone growth.

Pure 100% juices have some nutritional value, but their sugar content is so high it overshadows their value. Juices are *never* necessary, but as an alternative beverage for your child they are acceptable in moderation. Don't give juice to your infant and give your toddler only six to eight ounces a day.

Pop or soda is never a good choice for young children. They have absolutely *no* nutritional value. Pop fills up your child so they will have less appetite for healthy foods. The sugar content is a dental nightmare and the phosphorus content robs the bones of calcium by blocking its absorption. Pop is also expensive. Save it for an *occasional* treat for your older child only.

JUNK FOODS

With obesity becoming an epidemic among children, it is more important than ever to make good food choices. Consumption of large amounts of concentrated sweets (sugary foods and beverages) also contributes to the development of diabetes. It is essential to regulate the intake of these foods. Avoiding them completely makes them even more desirable, so teach your children to eat them in moderation as occasional treats.

Avoid fast food and junk food as much as possible. The fast food outlets target children with their give-away toys. Once hooked, your children will be their patron for life, eating foods high in fat and salt with much less nutritional value than more balanced meals prepared at home. Chips, crackers and the like are similarly high in fat and salt with proportionately less nutrition value. Try to find snacks for mid afternoon and after school with more food value, such as fruits and vegetables. Low fat pretzels are a good alternative to chips. You will help your children develop lifelong good eating habits.

- Make an effort to avoid foods with caffeine such as chocolate and colas. Some soft drinks are actually fortified with caffeine with the target audience being teenagers and young adults. Stay away from them yourself — be a good example!

Eating Disorders

The incidence of eating disorders is on the rise in adolescents and school age children.

Dr. Michael Eldredge rates healthy eating habits and weight control high on his list of priorities for children.

The unrealistic pictures presented in the media lead to body image concerns, especially in girls. Anorexia and bulimia may result as children and adolescents strive to achieve the bodies they think they should have. Our efforts must focus on prevention by education. A healthy weight — height ratio should be the goal. And, young people need to be comfortable with bodies that are right for them, not necessarily 'perfect' by the media's standards.

Be aware of your child's feelings about their body. Reinforce their positive attributes and build their self esteem and comfort with themselves. Encourage healthy eating habits rather than constantly saying "you shouldn't eat that, it's fattening," or "eat this we need to fatten you up."

In infancy and early childhood, children are excellent self regulators; they stop eating or push food away when they are full. It is important to read these cues in your child and not over feed them. Being a member of the 'clean plate club' is not always necessary and may be detrimental. Insist your children try everything and consume at least some of each food on their plate, but let them regulate their portions within reason.

Watch for signs of eating disorders in your older children. These may include refusing foods, moving food around on their plate, cutting food into tiny pieces and chewing for a long time, hoarding food, evidence of vomiting or purging (including diarrhea), discovery of laxatives or diet aids and evidence of excessive exercise. Obvious signs are significant weight loss, hair loss, overdressing, being cold all the time, and loss of enamel (staining) on the teeth.

Feeding your child seems so simple — but it's not. With all the pressures and risk factors parents have today, balanced eating is becoming one of the most difficult challenges we face. Remembering basic nutrition and moderation will be your best guides.

CHECKLIST

Use this Checklist to track your progress in meeting the recommendations in this chapter.

| Goal | Accomplished | | Will do | | By When |
	Yes	No	Yes	No	Date
Breast feed exclusively for the first several months					
Consume at least 450 calories extra (preferably 900) a day for optimum milk production					
No caffeine, alcohol or drugs while breastfeeding					
No smoking while breastfeeding					
Medicines only by prescription					
If you bottle feed, use a formula with iron					
Wait 4 to 6 months for solid food					
Establish regular meal times					
Whole cow's milk to age 2; 2% or less after that					
Limit juice intake					
No pop or soda					
Limit fast foods — high salt and fat content					
Avoid caffeine in colas and chocolate					
Your adolescent needs 1000 mg calcium per day					
Limit exposure to media which promotes an unrealistic body image in girls					
Watch for eating disorders					

Chapter 8
An Active Child
Is a Healthy Child

PLAY IS THE WORK of children. Activity helps them grow and develop and contributes to strong bones and muscles and a healthy weight.

PLAY TIME FOR BABY

Infants should have lots of 'floor time' so they can learn to roll over, crawl, pull up and, eventually, walk. 'Tummy time' is especially important since the implementation of the back lying sleep position. Babies need to be placed on their abdomens so they can learn to hold their heads and chests up and begin to scootch. 'Tummy time' also helps prevent flattening of the back of your baby's head. Remember to supervise your baby as he or she plays!

KEEP YOUR OLDER CHILD BUSY

Outdoor play for children is essential. As they grow, encourage them to be outside and to explore their environment. Children will find all sorts of things to play with and will use their imaginations outdoors, which stimulates their minds as well as their bodies. Children who are confined indoors for long periods of time can become cranky and unpleasant. So can their parents! We all need fresh air and physical activity to promote well-being. Take your child out into your yard or neighborhood park and play with them.

Children love to be around other children. This is evident beginning in infancy — they crave the attention of other children. If they don't have siblings, hook them up with playmates in your neighborhood or building. Find a play group within your community or start one. Encourage games and make believe and, again, remember to supervise. When your children are older look for group activities such as scouts or clubs.

Dr. Trent McNeeley encourages participation in church groups as a healthy outlet for social interaction.

When your child starts school they will participate in physical education classes and recess — reinforce this at home. Go on family walks or bicycle outings. Role model good physical activity for your children. Plan for regular physical activity outside of school at least three times a week after age 10. By then your child will be fairly independent, and physical education classes may no longer be required in the curriculum. Enroll your child in extracurricular activities after school if you are able. Dance, karate and gymnastics are some examples. Take them to a fitness center or gym and exercise together. Weight training for prepubertal children is not safe, but cardiovascular workouts (such as fast walking) are very beneficial. Keep in mind that nothing replaces good old unstructured play outdoors, whatever the season!

SPORTS PARTICIPATION

Organized competitive sports are a wonderful opportunity for your children to develop skills and to promote physical activity. Sports programs are available for children beginning in the preschool period — soccer, ice skating and hockey to name a few. As your child reaches school age they can play baseball, football, basketball, volleyball and other team sports. Golf and tennis can be lifelong physical activities — the earlier your child learns these skills, the more proficient they become. Organized sports teach discipline, group participation and accomplishment, and good health.

> *Cathy Carter has seen lots of evidence that sports participation is especially important for girls.*

Encouraging older elementary age girls towards sports will make them more likely to participate as teens. Older girls who are active in sports have higher grades and self esteem, and a lower incidence of eating disorders, depression, school absenteeism and teen pregnancy.

- Remember winning is fun, but playing is more important. Your attitude about sports will be communicated to your child. Teach them by your words and actions to be competitive and to do their best, but also to be a good sport and to have fun. **Don't try to make your child into a miniature adult who thinks winning is everything.** Children who learn this philosophy early become teenagers who take unnecessary risks such as rapid weight loss or performance enhancing drugs, or developing eating disorders, all of which can be deadly.

Regular physical activity is an essential part of a healthy lifestyle. Exercise reduces the risk of obesity, diabetes, hypertension and heart disease. Obesity and type II diabetes (the type previously associated with overweight adults) is becoming commonplace in children. The trend toward sedentary lifestyles (often in front of the TV or computer) in today's children will prove deadly. We must reverse this trend and get our children up, out, playing and exercising.

CHECKLIST

Use this Checklist to track your progress in meeting the recommendations in this chapter.

Goal	Accomplished		Will do		By When
	Yes	No	Yes	No	Date
Infants need floor time on their tummies					
Take your baby and child outside to play					
Find other children for play					
Look for scouts, church groups or clubs					
Plan family bicycling or outings					
Encourage after school activities — gymnastics, sports, karate, etc.					
Remember sports are a game and winning isn't everything					
Set a good example of sportsmanship					
Always supervise your child					

Chapter 9
You Are the Parent —
Act Like One

WHEN YOU BRING A NEW BABY into your home for the first time, it's a terrifying prospect. What if you 'do it wrong?' What if you 'wreck' your child? Shouldn't there be a 'license required' for something so important? There are only a few ingredients needed to make a good parent — love, commitment, common sense and patience. **Not all of parenting is fun. It's the hardest, but most rewarding work, you'll ever do.**

A MESSAGE

TO BRAND NEW MOTHERS

> *Dr. Paul Antal advises: "When you first bring your newborn home try to get enough sleep to be alert when your baby is awake."*

This will mean frequent naps because you won't be able to sleep for long stretches all at once. Get into the habit of bathing and dressing every day, even when you have been up most of the night and are exhausted — you will feel better. **You can't take care of**

your baby if you can't take care of yourself. Alternate care giving with the baby's father.

Find the time for regular meals and make sure the food you eat is nutritious and appealing. Family and friends may offer to help — take them up on it. You have to have strength to take care of your baby and this is especially so if you had a difficult delivery or a cesarean section. Remember, healing takes nourishment. If you are breastfeeding, and we hope you are, you need several hundred extra calories to provide nutritious breast milk without losing weight yourself (see chapter 1). Weight loss may be desirable, but it should be taken in context with the need to heal and to feed your baby.

As Your Child Grows

Dr. Michael Eldredge has seen evidence that the best parents "Set rules and limits and enforce them."

When your child becomes a toddler, you will need to set limits. At first they are about what to touch and what not to touch. Certainly, it's best to baby proof your home as we discussed in Chapter 3. Add to that the need to place knick knacks out of reach of your toddler — otherwise you will spend all your time picking up after them, rather than teaching limits. It's okay to say *'no'* rather forcefully. Try not to yell unless it's a real emergency (you will have one occasionally, and you will lose your temper), but do be firm. Your toddler will learn, because the one thing they want most is praise. So, when they do behave, be generous with your praise! Remember to be clear that you love them even if you don't like their behavior. You must not forget that children who seem to have learned all the rules will test to see if you are watching. "Parents need eyes in the back of their heads!" says Dr. Ward Griffen. When it becomes too quiet, go looking. You will learn as will your child.

When your child begins to play with brothers or sisters or other children, you will have to establish another set of rules. If all the children are yours, it's a little easier because you are the boss. With other people's children, it's a little more difficult. However, **you have the absolute right and duty to set rules in your house and yard.** Do it. Broadcast them. Enforce them. Children will respect you for that. When you allow your child to go to another house or yard to play, know the rules there. If they are not to your liking, negotiate with that parent or don't allow your child to go there. *You* make the choices for *your* children.

Set rules for bed time, nap time, meal time, play time, etc., and enforce them. The list is endless and continuously evolving. Don't be talked into violating one of your basic principles. Know where your children are at all times and with whom they are playing. Know what they are playing and what they are playing with. Sharp objects and guns are just as dangerous at someone else's house as they are at yours.

DISCIPLINE

Plan ahead the method of discipline you will use and be prepared to follow through. In the early years, 'time out' is very effective since **what your child craves most is your attention and approval.** The standard rule is one minute per year of age. So at 18 months it's a minute and a half which will seem like a lifetime to both you and your child. Remove them to a quiet place where they cannot see you and there is nothing to do — a specific chair, or the bottom step of a staircase. Avoid your child's bed, as you don't want to associate bed with punishment. The key is consistency, and both parents following through equally and *every time*. It can be exhausting, but necessary, to avoid sending mixed signals to your child.

When your child is older, loss of privileges or allowance money may be effective tools. Define what privileges are — perhaps TV or computer time, play time with friends, or a special activity. **Don't make threats you are unable or unwilling to follow through with.** It's very tempting in the heat of the moment!

- Make clear to your children what their limits are and the consequences for violating them. Make sure you and your mate present a united front so they can't play you off against one another. Don't be wishy-washy!
- It will be tempting to want to be your child's friend — it's hard to be the 'bad guy.' But keep this in mind — you *are* the parent, you *are* the grown-up, *you* have the authority and the power to help your child become the kind of person you want them to be. Don't miss your opportunity by being indifferent or too permissive.
- Remember, children are sponges. Make sure to role model only behavior you want to see again!

Privacy

As your child grows older, he or she will need some privacy, just as you do. They will need to learn to knock on doors before entering (especially to bathrooms and bedrooms). They will need to learn to respect the privacy of their brothers or sisters and in turn theirs must be respected (especially with regard to their rooms). This will become even more important as they go out into the world. Privacy is sacred for all of us and your children must learn to respect this basic rule. **But, as a parent, you must know where they are, what they are doing and with whom they are doing it.** They must earn and deserve your trust and you must also give them privacy, *unless* you have reason to question their safety.

Friends and

Other Outside Influences

Talk with your children about the people they surround themselves with. Stress the importance of not only having friends but having the *right* friends. We don't mean the 'right' friends in any artificial status situation. Rather, we mean 'right' in the sense of having a positive influence and the same values and morals you are trying to instill in your children. When your child announces a new friend, invite the friend to your house first where you can observe behavior before allowing a visit to the friend's house. Ask questions and try to meet the parents if you can arrange it.

It's better to be a little over protective than to end up being sorry.

Young teenagers looking for social acceptance and recognition may align themselves with other groups of teens with similar problems. Unfortunately, they seem to feed on each other, gaining support for their outcast position or lack of confidence. Even worse, the new group may be a gang. Gangs provide all sorts of support, but at a horrible price. Usually drugs, sex or other illegal activities are involved in the initiation process or in maintaining membership. Thievery and property destruction are common forms of acting out. Watch your teens. Pay attention to their friends. When they won't introduce you or discuss them, look out. Talk with the school counselor. Seek professional help if necessary. Explain the importance of morals, principles, values and aspirations. ***Above all,* demonstrate in your daily life what you mean. *They learn from you.***

Through all the challenges and ups and downs of your child's life, one thing remains constant — *you are the parent.* You will do your best only if you take your role seriously and unconditionally.

CHECKLIST

Use this Checklist to track your progress in meeting the recommendations in this chapter.

Goal	Accomplished Yes	No	Will do Yes	No	By When Date
Get enough sleep and take care of yourself in the newborn period					
Both parents should be involved care givers					
Toddlers need consistent limits					
Give praise generously when deserved					
Always let your child(ren) know you love them					
You make the rules for Your children					
Plan discipline and be prepared to follow through					
Time out is effective at 1 minute per year of age					
Set clear limits and consequences and implement them					
Remember — you can't avoid being a role model					
Teach your child about privacy					
Pay attention to your child's friends					
Be wary of friends your child won't discuss					

Chapter 10
Expand Your Horizons

IN A FAST PACED LIFE, it's tempting to focus only on the necessities such as feeding, bathing and the laundry. Intellectual and cultural stimulation for your child may be swept under the carpet as you go about the day-to-day tasks of life. Stimulating your child's brain is essential to their health and well being and it produces an intelligent well-rounded young adult.

INTERACT WITH YOUR BABY

Babies learn from their parents. Talk to them constantly as you care for them. Make eye contact and use facial expressions. Bath time and diaper changes are perfect opportunities for interaction. Use colorful mobiles and toys with many textures. Musical toys and ones with lights and sounds are wonderful choices. Board books can be introduced in early infancy. At first your baby will chew on them, but soon they will be looking at the pictures and colors. Read to your baby beginning in early infancy. Show your baby the pictures as you read the words.

READING IS FUN

Your toddler will be able to 'read' with you as they become familiar with the pictures. This is the first step toward reading. Choose a time each day to read with your child — bed time is a natural choice. Reading is a perfect component of a bed time settling routine. Soon, your older child will be reading to you. Help them sound out words and expand their vocabulary. Reading is an essential and lifelong skill. What a gift to give your child!

> *Dr. Trent McNeeley stresses that,*
> *"During the preschool and early school*
> *years, it is very important to see that*
> *intellectual stimulation... takes place."*

Your local public library and later your child's school library are excellent resources. Most public libraries have a story time for young children which will expose them to new books. It's entertaining — and free! The time with other children and adults at the library will enhance your child's learning and appreciation for reading. Utilize your public library for books at home, also. Purchase your favorites, but borrow others from the library because your child's interests and reading ability will change rapidly. Suggest books as gifts when relatives ask. They will be treasured items which can be passed on for generations.

MUSIC

Music is an integral part of life. Your baby will enjoy music beginning in infancy. Sing to them and play lullaby music quietly for them.

- Exposure to music has been shown in studies to increase children's math skills.
- Music can measurably lower stress levels in both children and adults.

Introduce your older children to many varieties of music so they will develop a well rounded attitude towards music in general. Be cautious with modern varieties as many of the lyrics are inappropriate for young ears. Violence, sex and drugs may be expressed subtly or overtly in the lyrics. CDs and tapes have a ratings system similar to that for movies. Make sure to check the rating before you buy. Some stores refuse to sell music which doesn't meet the rating designated for all audiences.

- Before playing any modern music for your child, listen to the lyrics yourself. Don't rely completely on the rating.
- Teach your older children your favorite songs and sing with them. Time in the car can be enjoyable when you're singing. Remember folk songs and historical songs. They're part of your heritage you'll want to pass on.

Enroll your child in music lessons (instrumental or vocal) if you are able. Lessons are often available through school.

TELEVISION

Television is a common and frequent presence in most homes. While watching TV can be informative and entertaining, it can also be addictive and expose children to issues which are not age-appropriate.

The American Academy of Pediatrics recommends no TV or video games for children under age two and no more than two hours a day of video exposure (including video and computer games) for children over the age of two.

While this may seem rigid, inappropriate TV exposure has been linked to an increase in violent behavior and desensitization to violence, to childhood obesity, and to an increase in promiscuous and precocious sexual behavior in children. Obviously parents need to interpret this recommendation in the way that fits the best in their household. Sometimes the TV can be a lifesaver to occupy your children while you accomplish household tasks. And, some TV shows and videos can be very educational for children, but too much of a good thing isn't always good.

- Try not to use TV as a babysitter except when absolutely necessary. It's an easy habit to start and very hard to break. Plan your TV time and choose programs carefully.
- *Always* watch any program, video or movie yourself before allowing your child to view it. Ratings systems are helpful, but be sure a program fits into your family's moral framework regardless of the rating.
- Don't be fooled by cartoons. Even the ones made when you were a child are among the most violent of programs.
- Be aware that commercials are geared to children and it can be very difficult to convince them that not all they see on TV is true.
- News programs may be informative, but horribly disturbing. It's hard for children to distinguish between events happening elsewhere and those happening in their own backyard. TV news can be upsetting for adults — doubly so for children.
- Don't ever think your children aren't paying attention when you are watching an adult program. They are hearing and absorbing every word. Save adult programming for after the children are asleep.

VIDEO GAMES

Video games have become a significant problem for children. What began as a fun pastime has evolved into an activity which consumes, distracts, and, as with some TV programs, promotes and desensitizes them to violence. Carefully screen your child's video games or choose not to allow them in your home. Know what happens in friend's homes. Again, don't rely on ratings — play the game yourself. Many video games are not meant for children.

- Some violent video games involving shooting and the use of a joystick are actually used in military training to desensitize soldiers to aiming and shooting at a target.

COMPUTERS

Computers are an amazing tool for business, organizational and educational purposes. Children have access to them in school, the library and often at home. It is important that parents decide which software is available and which games are played. Restrict access to the Internet while promoting learning to use a computer. Knowledge of computers is necessary now and will become even more so in the future. The convenience of access to information on the Internet is huge. However, it can be dangerous and frightening as well. Pornography is too easily accessed, connections can be made with criminals and other unscrupulous adults, and money can be spent in large amounts if your child has access to your credit card.

- Equip your computer with Internet filtering software to restrict access to websites inappropriate for children.
- Nothing substitutes for parental supervision. Monitor your children at all times when they are using the Internet.

Remember with *all* video — too much of a good thing is not good, even appropriate and "educational" choices in large doses can lead to problems. Encourage books and music as recreational choices.

CHECKLIST

Use this Checklist to track your progress in meeting the recommendations in this chapter.

Goal	Accomplished Yes	No	Will do Yes	No	By When Date
Talk to your baby					
Make faces and smile at your baby					
Read to your child					
Help your child read to you					
Use the library					
Suggest books as gifts					
Play background music					
Check the rating and listen to the lyrics before purchasing					
Sing with your child					
No TV or video games under age 2					
2 hours a day maximum for TV, video and computer over age 2					
Don't use TV as a baby sitter					
Delay news and adult programs until children are asleep					
Know what happens in friends' homes					
Use an Internet filter					

INDEX

For more information, contact:

Inside Advantage Publications
1240 Iroquois Drive, Suite 406
Naperville, IL 60563
Phone: 630.420.7673
Fax: 630.420.7835
rfritz3800@aol.com
http://www.rogerfritz.com

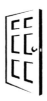